VITAMIN C, AND THEIR IMPORTANT TO HEALTH

Kristen J. Harris

1

Table of Contents

CHAPTER1

What is , or vitamin C,

Ascorbic acid, or vitamin C, is a water-soluble vitamin that can be found in many fruits and vegetables. Because it is a nutrient that our bodies cannot produce on their own, we must eat it because it is an essential nutrient. L-ascorbic acid has various significant capabilities in the body, for example, supporting the retention of iron, reinforcing the resistant framework, and going about as a cell reinforcement.

Collagen synthesis, the main protein in our bodies that gives our skin, bones, and muscles structure, is greatly aided by vitamin C. Additionally, it aids in the production of the molecule carnitine, which aids in the conversion of fat into energy. Furthermore, L-ascorbic acid is significant for the retention of iron, which is important for the creation of red platelets. It likewise goes about as a cancer prevention agent, shielding our cells from harm brought about by free extremists.

The suggested day to day admission of L-ascorbic acid fluctuates relying upon age, orientation, and wellbeing status. Adults should aim for 75-90 mg per day, with higher doses recommended for pregnant and breastfeeding women. Great wellsprings of L-ascorbic acid incorporate citrus organic products, strawberries, kiwi, mango, broccoli, spinach, and red and green ringer peppers. While L-ascorbic acid insufficiency is uncommon in evolved nations, it can prompt scurvy which is a lack of serious sickness described by weariness, shortcoming, and muscle torment. As a result, it's critical to consume enough vitamin C through a well-balanced diet or, if necessary, supplements.

L-ascorbic acid, otherwise called ascorbic corrosive, is a fundamental supplement that the body needs to appropriately work. It is a water-dissolvable nutrient, and that implies that it can't be put away in the body and should be renewed routinely through our eating regimen. L-ascorbic acid assumes a basic part in our general wellbeing, and its significance couldn't possibly be more significant.

CHAPTER2

Functions of Vitamin C's

Vitamin C's role as an antioxidant is one of its most important functions. Our bodies' cells are shielded from harm by free radicals thanks to antioxidants. Instable molecules called free radicals have the potential to harm cells and contribute to the onset of chronic conditions like arthritis, heart disease, and cancer. Vitamin C's protective effects are further enhanced by its role in the body's regeneration of other antioxidants, like vitamin E.

Vitamin C's role in the production of collagen is yet another important function. Skin, tendons, ligaments, and cartilage are all dependent on collagen, a protein. L-ascorbic acid is expected for the combination of collagen, and that truly intends that without sufficient degrees of nutrient

C, the body can't deliver sufficient collagen to keep up with the wellbeing of these tissues. This can cause joint pain, skin damage, and weakened blood vessels, among other health issues.

To summarize, vitamin C is an essential nutrient that is essential to our overall health. Its cancer prevention agent properties help to safeguard the body from harm brought about by free extremists, while its part in collagen creation is fundamental for keeping up with solid skin, ligaments, tendons, and ligament. Vitamin C, a water-soluble vitamin that plays a crucial role in maintaining the body's overall health, must be consumed in sufficient quantities for us to remain healthy. Fruits and vegetables like bell peppers, broccoli, spinach, citrus fruits, kiwis, and strawberries all contain this necessary nutrient. The immune system, which is in charge of shielding the body from diseases and infections, requires vitamin C to function properly. Sufficient admission of L-ascorbic acid can essentially support the insusceptible framework's capacity to ward off affliction and diseases.

The enhancement of one's immune system is one of the most common reasons for taking vitamin C supplements. Vitamin C is well-known for supporting the body's natural defenses and fighting infections. Certain individuals might take a day to day

L-ascorbic acid enhancement to assist with forestalling the normal cold or influenza, while others might take higher portions when they are feeling sickly. Additionally, taking vitamin C supplements may help shorten the duration and severity of respiratory infections like colds.

Vitamin C deficiency can occur for a variety of reasons. A lack of fruits and vegetables, which are the primary sources of vitamin C, in one's diet is one of the most common causes. People who consume a lot of processed foods and drinks may also be at risk of becoming deficient. Smoking, alcoholism, and certain medical conditions that affect the absorption and metabolism of vitamin C are additional contributors to a deficiency. People who are at risk for a vitamin C deficiency should think about taking supplements or increasing their intake of vitamin C-rich foods.

One of Vitamin C's most important benefits is that it is a potent antioxidant that helps protect our cells from free radical damage. Chronic conditions like cancer, heart disease, and arthritis can be brought on by oxidative stress, which is caused by unstable molecules called free radicals. These free radicals can't harm our cells because vitamin C can neutralize them.

Vitamin C has the additional advantage of strengthening our immune systems and assisting us in the fight against diseases and infections. L-ascorbic acid animates the creation of white platelets, which are answerable for fending off unfamiliar trespassers, like microscopic organisms and infections. Vitamin C can help lessen the severity and length of colds and flus, and it may even help prevent them from occurring in the first place, if consumed on a regular basis.

CHAPTER3

The methods and ways of vitamin C

There are several ways that vitamin C aids the immune system. First and foremost, it encourages the production of white blood cells, which are the ones in charge of preventing infections and other diseases. L-ascorbic acid additionally assists these white platelets with working all the more successfully by upgrading their capacity to annihilate destructive microorganisms, for example, infections and microscopic organisms. The production of antibodies, which are proteins that recognize, bind, and neutralize harmful toxins and pathogens, is also greatly aided by vitamin C. As a result, getting enough vitamin C is necessary to build a strong immune system that can effectively fight infections and diseases.

In addition, vitamin C is a potent antioxidant that aids in shielding cells from free radical damage. Instable molecules known as free radicals have the potential to cause oxidative stress, which in turn has the potential to harm cells and raise the risk of developing chronic conditions like arthritis, heart disease, and cancer. L-ascorbic acid kills these free extremists, diminishing the gamble of oxidative pressure and the related medical issues. Additionally, vitamin C's anti-inflammatory properties can aid in the body's reduction of inflammation, enhancing immune system function.

All in all, L-ascorbic acid is a fundamental supplement that assumes a vital part in keeping up with the general wellbeing of the body. Its capacity to advance the safe framework's capability and shield the cells from harm makes it a priceless supplement for keeping up with ideal wellbeing. As a result, those who may be deficient should take vitamin C supplements or eat a well-balanced diet to ensure adequate intake.

L-ascorbic acid is a fundamental supplement that is essential for our general wellbeing. Because it is a vitamin that dissolves in water and cannot be made by the body, we must consume it or take it in supplements. The essential capability of L-ascorbic acid is to go about as a cancer prevention agent, shielding our cells from free extreme harm. It is likewise fundamental for the creation of collagen, a protein that is tracked down in our skin, bones, and connective tissues.

Our skin's elasticity, firmness, and hydration are all essentially maintained by collagen, the body's most abundant protein. Our bodies produce less collagen as we get older, which causes wrinkles, sagging skin, and other signs of aging. Vitamin C plays a crucial role in this. A co-factor for the chemicals are liable for the blend of collagen. L-ascorbic acid assists with advancing collagen creation, which, thus, further develops skin wellbeing and diminishes the indications of maturing.

Vitamin C has been shown to boost collagen production in a number of studies. Women with better skin elasticity and fewer wrinkles were found to consume more Vitamin C, according to a study that was published in the American Journal of Clinical Nutrition. According to a different study that was published in the Journal of Investigative Dermatology, taking vitamin C supplements can help the skin produce more collagen. These examinations feature the significance of L-ascorbic acid in keeping up with sound skin and further developing collagen creation.

In conclusion, vitamin C is an essential nutrient for our overall health. Its job in collagen creation is especially significant for keeping up with solid skin, bones, and connective tissues. By advancing collagen creation, L-ascorbic acid can assist with further developing skin versatility, solidness, and hydration, prompting a more young appearance. To maintain optimal health, it is essential to ensure adequate intake of Vitamin C through diet or supplementation.

L-ascorbic acid is a fundamental supplement that is urgent for keeping up with great wellbeing. It is a vitamin that dissolves in water and cannot be made by the body; instead, we must get it from food or supplements. Vitamin C is well-known for its ability to improve skin and hair health, fight infections and inflammation, and strengthen the immune system. Additionally, it is an antioxidant that shields the body from free radicals, which have the potential to harm DNA and cells.

Consuming a variety of fruits and vegetables is one of the best ways to ensure that we are getting enough vitamin C in our diets. Vitamin C is abundant in citrus fruits like oranges, lemons, grapefruits, kiwis, mangoes, papayas, and strawberries. Vegetables, for example, broccoli, ringer peppers, and kale are additionally astounding wellsprings of L-ascorbic acid. It is essential to take note of that cooking can annihilate a portion of the L-ascorbic acid in these food varieties, so it is ideal to eat them crude or delicately cooked.

One more method for consolidating more L-ascorbic acid in our eating regimen is to add a L-ascorbic acid enhancement to our everyday daily practice. Supplements come in different structures, including tablets, powders, and chewy candies, and can be found all things considered wellbeing food stores. It is critical to follow the prescribed dose on the name and to talk with a medical services supplier prior to beginning any new enhancement routine. It is likewise critical to take note of that enhancements ought not be utilized as a substitute for a solid eating routine.

In conclusion, vitamin C is an essential nutrient that is essential for health maintenance. Consuming a variety of fruits and vegetables as well as, if necessary, taking a vitamin C supplement can help us consume more vitamin C. To ensure that we get all of the necessary nutrients for our bodies to function properly, it is essential to eat a well-balanced and healthy diet.

Vitamin C is a nutrient that is absolutely necessary for the body to function properly. Because it is a vitamin that dissolves in water and cannot be produced by the body, it must be obtained through diet or supplements. The suggested everyday admission of L-ascorbic acid for grown-ups is 75-90 mg each day. There are different wellsprings of L-ascorbic acid, both from plant and creature sources.

Vitamin C is mostly found in fruits and vegetables. Citrus fruits like oranges, lemons, limes, and grapefruit are well-known sources of vitamin C. Kiwi, strawberries, papaya, mango, and pineapple are also good sources of vitamin C. Vegetables, for example, broccoli, cauliflower, Brussels fledglings, and ringer peppers are likewise great wellsprings of L-ascorbic acid. Dull mixed greens like kale and spinach are additionally high in L-ascorbic acid.

Aside from leafy foods, a few creature sources likewise contain L-ascorbic acid. Liver and kidney of creatures, particularly the liver of cows and sheep, are plentiful in L-ascorbic acid. Nonetheless, it is fundamental for note that creature wellsprings of L-ascorbic acid don't give as much L-ascorbic acid as plant sources. In conclusion, vitamin C is an essential nutrient that is required for the proper functioning of the body. It is essential to note that food processing and cooking can destroy vitamin C. As a result, it is recommended to consume fresh fruits and vegetables to obtain the maximum benefits of vitamin C. It can come from a variety of things, like fruits, vegetables, and some animals. However, in order to reap the full benefits of vitamin C, fresh fruits and vegetables must be consumed. Vitamin C can be obtained by eating a well-balanced diet that includes a variety of fruits and vegetables. Vitamin C is an essential nutrient that is essential for maintaining good health.

Because it is a water-soluble vitamin, the body cannot make it, so it must be obtained through diet or supplements. One of the most incredible wellsprings of L-ascorbic acid is foods grown from the ground like oranges, kiwi, strawberries, broccoli, and chime peppers. Vitamin C, which supports the immune system, promotes healthy skin, and enhances iron absorption in the body, is abundant in these foods. L-ascorbic acid is additionally known for its cancer prevention agent properties, which help to shield cells from harm brought about by free revolutionaries.

CHAPTER4

Types of Vitamin C, fruits and their nutrients

Consuming sufficient L-ascorbic acid is fundamental for keeping up with great wellbeing. It is necessary for the growth and repair of the body's tissues as well as the healing of wounds. By encouraging the production of white blood cells, which aid in the fight against infection and disease, vitamin C also aids the immune system. It also plays a role in the production of collagen, a protein that is necessary for the skin, bones, and joints to be healthy.

Additionally, vitamin C is a potent antioxidant that contributes to the body's defense against oxidative stress and free radical damage.

Taking everything into account, L-ascorbic acid is a significant supplement that is fundamental for keeping up with great wellbeing. It can be obtained through supplements as well as in a variety of foods, including fruits and vegetables. Vitamin C is essential for supporting the immune system, promoting skin health, and enhancing iron absorption in the body. It also plays a role in the production of collagen and has antioxidant properties that aid in the body's defense against free radical damage. Thusly, it is vital to remember L-ascorbic acid rich food sources for your eating routine to guarantee that you are getting enough of this fundamental supplement.

Vitamin C, an essential nutrient that aids in immune system health, encourages tissue growth and repair, and serves as an antioxidant, can be found in abundance in fruits. Oranges, strawberries, kiwis, papaya, guava, and pineapple are a few examples of vitamin C-rich fruits. These natural products can be polished off in their regular structure or as juices, smoothies, or mixed greens.

One of the most widely consumed fruits, oranges are well-known for their high vitamin C content. One enormous orange contains around 70 milligrams of L-ascorbic acid, which is more than the suggested everyday admission for grown-ups. Also, strawberries are one more magnificent wellspring of L-ascorbic acid, with only one cup of new strawberries giving over 100 percent of the everyday suggested admission of this supplement.

Another fruit with a lot of Vitamin C is the kiwi, which has about 70 milligrams of this nutrient per medium-sized kiwi. One medium-sized papaya and one medium-sized guava each contain approximately 100 milligrams and 125 milligrams of Vitamin C, respectively. Last but not least, one cup of fresh pineapple chunks contains approximately 80 milligrams of the vitamin C that is found in pineapple, a tropical fruit.

In general, eating a variety of fruits with a lot of Vitamin C is a great way to make sure your body gets the nutrients it needs to be at its best. Organic products give L-ascorbic acid, yet additionally other fundamental nutrients, minerals, and fiber that are significant for keeping a sound eating regimen. Integrating these natural products into your eating regimen can assist you with meeting your everyday supplement necessities and backing your general wellbeing and prosperity.

Vitamin C is a water-soluble vitamin that is necessary for the body to function properly. It is fundamental for the development and fix of tissues, the arrangement of collagen, and the retention of iron. While L-ascorbic acid is ordinarily connected with citrus organic products, there are various vegetables that are additionally incredible wellsprings of this supplement.

Vitamin C is abundant in vegetables, and many of them contain even higher concentrations than citrus fruits. For instance, ringer peppers are an especially decent wellspring of L-ascorbic acid, with one medium-sized pepper giving around 150% of the suggested everyday admission. Different vegetables that are high in L-ascorbic acid incorporate broccoli, Brussels fledglings, kale, and cauliflower. Vegetables can lose their vitamin C content when cooked, but steaming or lightly sautéing them can help keep their nutrients intact.

CHAPTER5

Integrating L-ascorbic acid rich vegetables into your eating routine can be an extraordinary method for guaranteeing that you are getting enough of this fundamental supplement. You can have a go at adding ringer peppers, broccoli, or kale to your servings of mixed greens, or broiling cauliflower or Brussels sprouts as a delectable side dish. By rolling out these straightforward improvements to your eating regimen, you can receive the many rewards of L-ascorbic acid, including worked on insusceptible capability, better skin, and a decreased gamble of constant infection.

Because it plays a crucial role in repairing tissues, supporting the immune system, and facilitating the absorption of iron, vitamin C is an essential nutrient for maintaining a healthy body. While L-ascorbic acid can be found in various food sources, certain individuals might decide to take L-ascorbic acid enhancements to guarantee they are getting enough of this fundamental supplement. Tablets, capsules, and powders are all possible forms of vitamin C supplements.

Supporting skin health is yet another reason why people may choose to take Vitamin C supplements. L-ascorbic acid is a strong cell reinforcement that can help safeguard against sun harm and advance collagen creation, which can further develop skin flexibility and diminish the presence of barely recognizable differences and kinks. A few investigations have likewise recommended that L-ascorbic acid enhancements might assist with decreasing the gamble of skin disease. However, it is essential to keep in mind that, despite the fact that vitamin C supplements may be beneficial to skin health, they should not be used in place of sunscreen or other measures to protect against the sun.

By and large, L-ascorbic acid enhancements can be a helpful and compelling method for guaranteeing that your body is getting enough of this fundamental supplement. However, it is essential to seek the advice of a medical professional before beginning any new supplements because some people may experience adverse effects from taking excessive amounts of vitamin C. In addition, it is essential to keep in mind that despite the fact that supplements can be beneficial, they should not be used in place of a diet that is both healthy and well-balanced. Eating different foods grown from the ground that are plentiful in L-ascorbic acid is as yet the most ideal way to guarantee that your body is getting every one of the supplements it necessities to remain sound.

Vitamin C is a nutrient that our bodies need in small amounts to do a number of important things. It is a vitamin that dissolves in water and is also referred to as ascorbic acid. As a result, our bodies are unable to store it, so we must consume it. A lack of L-ascorbic acid can prompt a few medical conditions, including scurvy. A condition known as scurvy is brought on by a prolonged lack of vitamin C in the diet. It is described by side effects like weariness, shortcoming, muscle and joint torment, and draining gums.

The most effective way to forestall a L-ascorbic acid insufficiency is to keep a sound and adjusted diet that incorporates a lot of foods grown from the ground. Citrus fruits, strawberries, kiwis, tomatoes, bell peppers, and broccoli are among the best sources of vitamin C. Fruits and vegetables should be eaten raw or lightly cooked because cooking and processing can lower vitamin C levels. Consider taking vitamin C supplements if you cannot get enough from your diet. In any case, it is essential to counsel a medical services proficient prior to beginning any enhancements to guarantee that they are protected and viable for you.

L-ascorbic acid, otherwise called ascorbic corrosive, is a water-dissolvable nutrient that assumes a significant part in different physical processes. It is fundamental for the development and fix of tissues in the body, including bones, skin, and veins. Additionally, vitamin C is a potent antioxidant that contributes to the body's defense against free radical damage. Additionally, it helps make collagen, a protein that keeps skin, cartilage, and tendons healthy.

One of the main elements of L-ascorbic acid is its capacity to help the invulnerable framework. White blood cells, which are responsible for fighting infections and diseases, are stimulated by it. L-ascorbic acid is additionally essential for the assimilation of iron from plant-based food sources, which is significant for the anticipation of pallor. Also, L-ascorbic acid is engaged with the development of synapses, which are synthetic couriers that send signals in the cerebrum. Additionally, it is thought to possess anti-inflammatory properties that may assist in lowering the risk of chronic conditions like arthritis, cancer, and heart disease.

Maintaining adequate levels of vitamin C in the body is crucial due to its significance. Notwithstanding, lacks in L-ascorbic acid can happen because of different variables, including less than stellar eating routine, liquor abuse, smoking, and certain ailments. Side effects of L-ascorbic acid insufficiency incorporate weariness, shortcoming, joint agony, and draining gums. On the other hand, taking too much vitamin C can result in vitamin C overdose, which can cause stomach cramps, nausea, and diarrhea. Therefore, for optimal health, it is essential to consume vitamin C in a balanced manner

L-ascorbic acid is a fundamental supplement that our body expects to appropriately work. A water-dissolvable nutrient is tracked down in many leafy foods. Despite its significance, our bodies are unable to produce Vitamin C on their own, so we must consume it from food. L-ascorbic acid insufficiency is a typical issue that can prompt numerous medical problems.

CHAPTER6

Signs and side effects of L-ascorbic acid

The signs and side effects of L-ascorbic acid insufficiency can change contingent upon the seriousness of the inadequacy. Fatigue, weakness, and irritability are the most common symptoms. Individuals who are lacking in L-ascorbic acid may likewise encounter joint and muscle throbs, enlarged and draining gums, and slow twisted recuperating. Vitamin C deficiency can, in severe cases, cause scurvy, a disease that causes gum disease, joint pain, and skin rashes.

A diet high in vitamin C is essential to avoid vitamin C deficiency. Fruits like oranges, strawberries, and kiwis are excellent sources of vitamin C, as are vegetables like broccoli, spinach, and bell peppers. Supplements may be required if a person cannot get enough Vitamin C from their diet. However, because taking too much vitamin C can result in an overdose, it is essential to seek medical advice before taking any supplements.

All in all, L-ascorbic acid insufficiency is a typical issue that can prompt numerous medical problems. Vitamin C deficiency can manifest as anything from fatigue and weakness to severe gum disease and skin rashes. Vitamin C deficiency can be prevented by eating a diet high in vitamin C. If a person cannot get enough vitamin C from their diet, they may need to take vitamin C supplements, but it is important to talk to a doctor before doing so to avoid overdosing.

A nutrient that is absolutely necessary for our bodies to function properly is vitamin C.

numerous vegetables and fruits contain it, which is a vitamin that dissolves in water. Despite its significance, our bodies are unable to produce Vitamin C on their own, so we must consume it from food. A common problem that can result in a variety of health issues is vitamin C deficiency.

Depending on the severity of the deficiency, vitamin C deficiency can present with a variety of symptoms. Fatigue, weakness, and irritability are the most common symptoms. Individuals who are lacking in L-ascorbic acid may likewise encounter joint and muscle throbs, enlarged and draining gums, and slow twisted mending. Vitamin C deficiency can, in severe cases, cause scurvy, a disease that causes gum disease, joint pain, and skin rashes.

A diet high in vitamin C is essential to avoid vitamin C deficiency. Fruits like oranges, strawberries, and kiwis are excellent sources of vitamin C, as are vegetables like broccoli, spinach, and bell peppers. Supplements may be required if a person cannot get enough Vitamin C from their diet. Be that as it may, it is essential to counsel a specialist prior to taking any enhancements, as unreasonable measures of L-ascorbic acid can prompt excess.

All in all, L-ascorbic acid insufficiency is a typical issue that can prompt numerous medical problems. Vitamin C deficiency can manifest as anything from fatigue and weakness to severe gum disease and skin rashes. Vitamin C deficiency can be prevented by eating a diet high in vitamin C. If a person cannot get enough vitamin C from their diet, they may need to take vitamin C supplements, but it is important to talk to a doctor before doing so to avoid overdosing.

CHAPTER 7

How can Vitamin C deficiency acid, prompt different medical issues.

One of the essential vitamins that the body needs to function properly is vitamin C. Lack of this nutrient can prompt a few unexpected issues and can meaningfully affect the body. The essential capability of L-ascorbic acid is to help the safe framework and advance the development and improvement of tissues all through the body. In the event that the body doesn't get satisfactory measures of L-ascorbic acid, it can prompt different medical issues.

The outcomes of L-ascorbic acid insufficiency can be extreme and can influence the body in more than one way. Scurvy is one of the most common signs of vitamin C deficiency. Joint pain, dry, scaly skin, and swollen, bleeding gums are all symptoms of scurvy. Different side effects of L-ascorbic acid insufficiency incorporate exhaustion, shortcoming, and frailty. L-ascorbic acid insufficiency can likewise prompt a debilitated insusceptible framework, making the body more defenseless to contaminations and sicknesses.

Vitamin C deficiency can pose particular dangers to particular populations. For instance, individuals who smoke, have a terrible eating routine, or have specific ailments, like Crohn's illness, are at a higher gamble of L-ascorbic acid insufficiency. Pregnant ladies and breastfeeding moms likewise require higher measures of L-ascorbic acid than the typical individual. Vitamin C deficiency can cause serious health problems, so it's critical to make sure you get enough of it through food or supplements.

Vitamin C, also known as ascorbic acid, is a necessary nutrient that is essential to good health. It is necessary for the immune system to function properly and for body tissues to grow, develop, and be repaired. However, as with any other nutrient, vitamin C overconsumption can result in an overdose with severe consequences. L-ascorbic acid excess happens when a singular takes a lot of the supplement than the body's day to day necessity.

A condition known as hypervitaminosis C, which can cause nausea, diarrhea, abdominal pain, and headaches, can be caused by taking too much vitamin C. It can also result in kidney stones, which can be painful and uncomfortable in severe cases. Hypervitaminosis C happens when a singular takes in excess of 2000 mg of L-ascorbic acid each day, which is well over the suggested day to day admission of 75-90 mg for grown-ups.

It is fundamental for note that L-ascorbic acid excess is interesting, and the vast majority can consume elevated degrees of the supplement without encountering any antagonistic impacts. Be that as it may, people who take L-ascorbic acid enhancements or eat sustained food sources ought to be wary and not surpass the suggested everyday admission. In general, although vitamin C is necessary for good health, it is essential to consume it in moderation to avoid any adverse effects that may result from consuming too much of it. Before taking any supplements, it is advisable to consult a healthcare provider to ensure that you are not consuming an excessive amount of any nutrient, including vitamin C.

Vitamin C is a nutrient that is absolutely necessary for our bodies to function properly. A cancer prevention agent assists with safeguarding our cells from harm brought about by free extremists. It likewise supports the creation of collagen, which is important for sound skin, hair, and nails. While it is essential to consume sufficient L-ascorbic acid, it is similarly critical to know about the dangers and side effects of L-ascorbic acid excess.

Vitamin C overdose can result in a number of risks and symptoms. Diarrhea is one of the most common side effects of vitamin C overdose. This is due to the fact that vitamin C dissolves in water and is excreted in excess through urine. Nausea, vomiting, stomach cramps, headaches, and insomnia are additional signs of vitamin C overdose. Vitamin C overdose can occasionally result in more serious health issues like iron overload and kidney stones.

It is essential to consume the daily dose of vitamin C that is recommended for adults, which ranges from 75 to 90 milligrams, in order to avoid the dangers of vitamin C overdose. This can be gotten through a fair eating routine that incorporates leafy foods like oranges, kiwis, broccoli, and chime peppers. It is likewise essential to know about the L-ascorbic acid substance of enhancements and to try not to take more than the suggested measurement. It is advised that you consult a medical professional if you experience any signs of vitamin C overdose.

Vitamin C is an essential nutrient that is required by the body for a variety of functions, including wound healing, infection prevention, and skin health maintenance. Nonetheless, similar to some other supplement, consuming L-ascorbic acid in moderation is fundamental. Over the top admission of L-ascorbic acid can prompt different unfortunate results that can be adverse to one's wellbeing.

Having a high intake of vitamin C can have a significant impact on digestive health. There is a risk of stomach cramps, nausea, and diarrhea when taking in large quantities of vitamin C. The body is unable to absorb all of the excess Vitamin C, which builds up in the intestines and causes these symptoms. This collection can disturb the covering of the stomach and cause these awkward side effects.

One more outcome of unnecessary L-ascorbic acid admission is the development of kidney stones. Vitamin C is eliminated from the body through urine, and excessive consumption can cause oxalate crystals in the kidneys. These crystals have the potential to get bigger, leading to kidney stones, which can be very painful and uncomfortable. In addition, to avoid any complications, individuals who have a history of kidney stones should consume Vitamin C with extreme caution.

Last but not least, taking too much vitamin C can be bad for your immune system. Vitamin C is known to strengthen the immune system, but taking too much of it can have the opposite effect. Consuming too much vitamin C can suppress the immune system, making the body more susceptible to illnesses and infections. To avoid negative effects, vitamin C consumption in moderation is essential.

All in all, while L-ascorbic acid is fundamental for generally wellbeing and prosperity, consuming it in moderation is urgent. Consuming too much vitamin C can have a number of negative effects, including problems with the digestive system, kidney stones, and lowered immunity. As a result, people should talk to a doctor or other medical professional to find out how much Vitamin C they need every day and how to avoid any potential side effects. By consuming L-ascorbic acid with some restraint, indiviuals can guarantee ideal wellbeing and prosperity.

L-ascorbic acid is a fundamental supplement that assumes a basic part in keeping our body solid. It is also involved in the production of collagen, a protein that keeps our skin, bones, and teeth healthy. It is an antioxidant that protects our body from harmful free radicals. However, vitamin C needs to be balanced in our bodies in the same way that other vitamins do, as both deficiencies and overdoses can be harmful to our health.

Vitamin C deficiency can be avoided relatively easily. The simplest method for forestalling an inadequacy is to guarantee that you are consuming sufficient L-ascorbic acid through your eating regimen. L-ascorbic acid is found in many foods grown from the ground, including citrus natural products, strawberries, kiwi, mangoes, papayas, tomatoes, ringer peppers, and broccoli. Consider taking a vitamin C supplement if your diet does not provide you with sufficient vitamin C. The treatment for vitamin C overdose is to simply stop taking any supplements or consuming foods that are high in vitamin C. Symptoms of vitamin C overdose may include diarrhea, nausea, and stomach cramps. However, it is important to be cautious when taking supplements because it is possible to overdose on vitamin C. However, it is essential to keep in mind that consuming a diet alone makes it extremely difficult to overdose on vitamin C. The body can flush out abundance L-ascorbic acid through pee, so it is improbable that you will encounter any adverse consequences from eating a lot of L-ascorbic acid through food alone.

In conclusion, vitamin C is an essential nutrient that contributes significantly to our overall health. Since both overconsumption and deficiency of vitamin C can be harmful to our health, it is critical that our bodies maintain a healthy balance. To forestall a lack, it is essential to consume sufficient L-ascorbic acid through your eating routine or think about taking an enhancement if important. Vitamin C is an essential nutrient that plays a crucial role in many physiological processes in our body. If you are experiencing symptoms of an overdose of vitamin C, it is important to stop taking any supplements or consuming foods that are high in vitamin C. It supports the immune system, contributes to the production of collagen, and serves as an antioxidant. Notwithstanding, it is essential to take note of that both lack and go too far of L-ascorbic acid can prompt antagonistic wellbeing impacts. L-ascorbic acid insufficiency can prompt scurvy, a condition that causes exhaustion, joint torment, and draining gums. As a result, it's critical to take the necessary precautions to avoid vitamin C deficiency.

Including foods high in vitamin C in your diet is one of the best ways to prevent vitamin C deficiency. Vitamin C can be found in a variety of citrus fruits, including grapefruits, oranges, lemons, and grapefruit, as well as kiwis, strawberries, and pineapple. Vegetables like broccoli, ringer peppers, and tomatoes are additionally great wellsprings of L-ascorbic acid. Remembering these food varieties for your day to day diet can assist you with meeting your everyday L-ascorbic acid prerequisites.

CHAPTER8

Avoid certain lifestyle practices

Avoiding certain lifestyle practices that can hinder your body's ability to absorb vitamin C is another way to prevent vitamin C deficiency. Smoking and drinking can make it harder for the body to absorb vitamin C. Subsequently, in the event that you are in danger of lack, keeping away from these propensities or breaking point their utilization to a minimum is ideal. In addition, it is essential to discuss this with your doctor and take the necessary precautions if you are taking any medications that can reduce vitamin C absorption.

In conclusion, vitamin C is a vital nutrient that is essential for health maintenance. To forestall lack, it is essential to remember L-ascorbic acid rich food sources for your everyday eating routine and stay away from way of life propensities that can decrease the assimilation of this supplement in your body. You can ensure that your body receives sufficient Vitamin C to support its various functions by taking these necessary steps.

Vitamin C is an essential nutrient that is very important for keeping your health good. A water-dissolvable nutrient can't be put away in the body, so it should be drunk consistently through food or enhancements. Age, gender, and other factors influence the amount of vitamin C that should be consumed on a daily basis. For most grown-ups, the suggested day to day admission is somewhere in the range of 75 and 90 milligrams each day. However, depending on their health and lifestyle, some people may require more or less.

It is essential to take note of that consuming an excess of L-ascorbic acid can prompt unfriendly wellbeing impacts. As far as possible for everyday admission of L-ascorbic acid is 2,000 milligrams each day for most grown-ups. Consuming beyond what this sum can cause gastrointestinal aggravations like loose bowels, sickness, and stomach cramps. High vitamin C intake can occasionally result in kidney stones and other serious health issues. In this way, it is essential to keep the protected admission rules for L-ascorbic acid to stay away from any bad wellbeing impacts.

When it comes to safe vitamin C intake guidelines, it is always preferable to get your daily dose from food rather than from supplements. L-ascorbic acid can be found in various products of the soil, for example, citrus organic products, strawberries, kiwi organic product, broccoli, chime peppers, and tomatoes. Including a variety of these foods in a well-balanced diet can guarantee that you get the vitamin C you need every day. Nonetheless, in the event that you can't get sufficient L-ascorbic acid from food, taking an enhancement might be fundamental. Before taking any vitamin C supplements, it is important to talk to a doctor to make sure you are taking the right amount for your needs.

A vital nutrient for our overall health and well-being, vitamin C is an essential nutrient. A water-solvent nutrient assumes a vital part in the development and fix of tissues in our body. While many people are aware that vitamin C can help prevent scurvy, few are aware of the additional advantages it offers to our health and well-being.

At last, L-ascorbic acid is fundamental for the creation of collagen, a protein that is vital for the development and fix of our skin, bones, and connective tissues. Our skin's elasticity and youthful appearance are both provided by collagen. Vitamin C can help improve the appearance of scars and stretch marks, as well as help prevent wrinkles, sagging skin, and other signs of aging.

L-ascorbic acid is a fundamental supplement that assumes a significant part in keeping up with great wellbeing. A water-dissolvable nutrient goes about as a cancer prevention agent, assisting with safeguarding cells from harm brought about by free extremists. L-ascorbic acid likewise assumes a vital part in the creation of collagen, which is a urgent part of skin, bones, and connective tissues. Additionally, it boosts the immune system, making it better able to fight off diseases and infections.

A variety of health issues, including scurvy, which is characterized by fatigue, weakness, and bleeding gums, can result from vitamin C deficiency. Dry skin, prolonged wound healing, and impaired immune function are additional signs of vitamin C deficiency. To avoid these health issues, it's important to make sure your diet contains enough vitamin C. Broccoli, kiwi, citrus fruits, and strawberries are all sources of vitamin C.

While L-ascorbic acid is significant for good wellbeing, ingesting too much this nutrient is additionally conceivable. Taking a lot of L-ascorbic acid can prompt stomach upset, the runs, and queasiness. It may even result in kidney stones or other serious health issues in some instances. It is essential to keep suggested everyday admission rules for L-ascorbic acid and to try not to take huge dosages of enhancements without first counseling a medical services proficient. By keeping a decent eating regimen and observing suggested rules, you can guarantee that you are getting sufficient L-ascorbic acid to keep up with great wellbeing without gambling an excess.

In conclusion, it is essential to consume Vitamin C in moderation because deficiency can result in serious health problems like scurvy, which can cause weakness, fatigue, and even death. However, taking too much Vitamin C can also cause problems with the digestive system, kidney stones, and problems with the body's ability to absorb other essential vitamins and minerals.

Adults should consume 75-90 milligrams of vitamin C daily, but this can vary based on age, gender, and other factors. It is vital to help this supplement through entire food varieties like products of the soil, instead of depending exclusively on supplements. This guarantees that the body receives a variety of other essential nutrients.

In conclusion, despite the fact that vitamin C is a necessary nutrient for good health, it is essential to strike a healthy balance and avoid overconsuming it. A sound eating routine comprising of different leafy foods can give sufficient measures of L-ascorbic acid, and enhancements ought to just be taken under the direction of a medical care proficient. By being aware of our L-ascorbic acid admission, we can forestall inadequacies and stay away from the adverse consequences of going too far.

THE   END